Flavio Freinkel Rodrigues
Eliete B. Cardoso
Joana A. Donzelli

Congenital Malformations of the Central Nervous System

Flavio Freinkel Rodrigues
Eliete B. Cardoso
Joana A. Donzelli

Congenital Malformations of the Central Nervous System

Neural Tube Defects - Embryonic, surgical, socioeconomic and psychological aspects

ScienciaScripts

Imprint
Any brand names and product names mentioned in this book are subject to trademark, brand or patent protection and are trademarks or registered trademarks of their respective holders. The use of brand names, product names, common names, trade names, product descriptions etc. even without a particular marking in this work is in no way to be construed to mean that such names may be regarded as unrestricted in respect of trademark and brand protection legislation and could thus be used by anyone.

Cover image: www.ingimage.com

This book is a translation from the original published under ISBN 978-613-9-69695-6.

Publisher:
Sciencia Scripts
is a trademark of
Dodo Books Indian Ocean Ltd. and OmniScriptum S.R.L publishing group

120 High Road, East Finchley, London, N2 9ED, United Kingdom
Str. Armeneasca 28/1, office 1, Chisinau MD-2012, Republic of Moldova, Europe
Printed at: see last page
ISBN: 978-620-7-77328-2

Thank you.

Maternidade Escola da UFRJ for supporting our research activities, especially Prof. Dr. Joffre Amim Jr. for sparing no effort to help with our project.

" child at the UFRJ Maternity Hospital to Prof. Dr. Marisa Shargel Maya and Prof. Marcus Renato de Carvalho for opening the doors for the development of scientific work.

We would like to express our great gratitude to Dr. Cesar Fantesia Andraus for his help in field activities and research support.

SUMMARY

I. INTRODUCTION

Myelomeningocele is the most complex of all CNS congenital malformations, compatible with prolonged survival, combined with spinal, brain, peripheral nerve, and osteoarticular anomalies. Contrary to what one might assume, a large number of people with the defect have normal or near-normal intellectual quotient.

Analysis of the natural course of cystic spinal cleft shows that most fatal complications occur during the first year of life, most of them associated with signs and symptoms of bulbo-cervical junction lesions resulting from Chiari malformation type II. (MCLONE DG, 1992).

Surgical treatment of neonates with myelomeningocele has long been the subject of debate because of poor outcomes and poor prognosis. Since 1970, with the advent of more effective valve systems for the treatment of hydrocephalus, the most serious complication, indications began to focus on early treatment of myelomeningocele, demonstrating that correction within the first 24 hours after birth offers a good chance of improvement. in motor prognosis. (PERRY and Coles, 2002).

Most children with myelomeningocele (80-85%) develop hydrocephalus requiring a liquor shunt, with the need for shunting being greater the higher the focus of the lesion. (ZAMBELLI and MALDAUM, 2009).

Myelomeningocele is a disease whose incidence in the population remains constant despite efforts to prevent it. In 1970, the mortality rate was close to 100%; current medical advances and the possibility of early neurosurgical intervention and urologic treatment to avoid renal complications have increased the mortality rate to about 12-20%. Prenatal ultrasound diagnosis of malformation is essential and reaches 100% in tertiary centers, but accurate determination of the level of the lesion is still a barrier to prognosis. Prognosis is directly related to the level of injury and the presence of ventriculomegaly. IQ for lower level defects is normal, as is the ability to walk. (BERNARDES et al., 2006).

Neural tube closure defects are important determinants of perinatal morbidity and mortality. All children with anencephaly are stillborn or die shortly after birth. Children with meningocele and myelomeningocele have a higher survival rate, usually due to extensive medical treatment and surgical management. The risk of death depends on the severity of the injury and other factors such as the availability of medical and surgical resources. Latent spinal cleft can progress asymptomatically throughout life.

Regarding the epidemiologic aspect of this malformation, three different types have been clinically described: the 1st group is prevalent among Celtic descendants, a high degree of lesion accompanied by mental retardation; the 2nd group predominates in persons of Spanish race and Arab origin, with good motor function and minimal mental retardation; the third group is formed among people of Sikh race living in western Canada, neurologic function is preserved in these patients.

The mean incidence of myelomeningocele ranges from 0.7 to 0.8 per 1000 live births with variation between regions: England 0.7 to 2.5 per 1000 live births; USA 0.41 to 1.43 per 1000 live births; Africans 0.1 per 1000 live births; Continental Europe: 0.41 to 1.9 per 1000 live births. (DIAS MS; MCLONE DG 2008).

In Brazil, according to the National Information System DATASUS, in 2016, a total of 2,857,800 births occurred, of which 4,085 were born with congenital malformations of the central nervous system, with 735 cases of cleft spine. In the city of Rio de Janeiro, out of 89,480 live births, 960 were born with congenital anomalies of the central nervous system, described statistically, highlighting cases of cleft spine, which accounted for a total of 30 (BRAZIL, 2017).

Central nervous system malformations are not the most common in statistical terms, but their consequences represent a large social impact; which has led to significant changes in the family nucleus of these patients. Congenital malformations may be a consequence of the living and health conditions of certain groups in society. (MELLO et al., 1993).

A child with a menigocele or myelomeningocele may have severe chronic disorders such as limb paralysis, hydrocephalus, limb and spinal deformities, bladder, bowel and sexual dysfunction, and learning difficulties, with a risk of psychosocial maladjustment .

In the United States, the lifetime cost of each child born with a cleft spine is estimated at approximately $294,000. The public health costs here in Brazil for these patients are high, as they require the assistance of several specialists and long-term treatment. In our system, the lack of public policies regarding these specific cases, in many cases, makes treatment difficult and inaccessible for families. as they move between several institutions, requiring constant care and high costs.

Because of the severity of neural tube closure defects and their high morbidity and mortality, genetic counseling, folic acid supplementation, and prenatal diagnosis of these malformations are very important.

Early diagnosis of congenital malformations of the central nervous system can significantly affect the survival and quality of life of the newborn; favoring intervention with a better prognosis. This can be done through ultrasound during pregnancy and measurement of alpha-fetoprotein in the amniotic fluid, values of which will be elevated through amniocentesis between $14^{и}$ 16 $^{\text{weeks of}}$ gestation. (AGIAR. MJB 2003).

A large number of imprecise terms contribute to confusion in naming neural tube closure defects. Spinal dysraphism includes all forms of spinal cleft, although the term is used by many specialists for both myelomeningocele and other spinal dysraphisms. The classification of spinal dysraphisms divides these malformations into two categories: open (open spinal cleft) and closed (hidden spinal cleft). Open forms of spinal dysraphism are characterized by impaired development of the skin, defects in bones, brain membranes, and nervous tissue, which leads to a disruption of communication of the lesion with the external environment.

Closed forms of dysraphism are anomalies in which there is a midline closure defect, malformations of bone and nerve tissue, but with preserved skin, although some dysraphisms are combined with skin anomalies. Skin lesions include lipomas, hemangiomas, skin patches, lipomeningomyelocele, terminal filament lipoma, dermoid and epidermoid cysts, and dermal sinus. These injuries are often diagnosed in childhood, but symptoms may not appear until years later.

Prenatal diagnosis is based on the measurement of alpha-fetoprotein in maternal serum at the beginning of the second trimester. A high level of alpha-fetoprotein compared to maternal age is a predictor of a high probability of neural tube closure defect. It should be considered that a large number of other congenital anomalies can also cause an increase in maternal serum alpha-fetoprotein. In these cases, ultrasound should be done in the second trimester of pregnancy. Prenatal ultrasound can detect the level of injury (in about two-thirds of patients), as well as the presence of lower limb deformities and other associated anomalies such as Chiari II and hydrocephalus.

During pregnancy, parents construct idealized images about the child who will be born. According to Brazelton and Kramer (1992), paternal representations come into play at the time of birth: the 'imaginary child, the fantasy child, and the real child will occupy the parents. ' Mind. When parents realize that the real child is different from the imaginary child, they undergo an intense process of adjustment and the formation of an emotional bond may be disrupted, especially when the newborn (NB) has a malformation.

The bond between parents and infants is gradually built starting from the prenatal period, according to some authors (Lebovici, 1987; Brazelton & Cramer, 1992), numerous factors influence the formation of the bond between parents and children, among them we can mention the parents' history. life, parents' perceptions, child characteristics, family and social context. Each birth causes major changes in the parents' life and personality. The dimensions of values change and the places each family member occupies are rearranged according to the birth of a new child. A wide variety of feelings arise and occupy the domestic scene. But when the unborn child has a congenital malformation, parents experience feelings of despair and longing, and depending on the severity of the condition, parents may have difficulty in the process of emotionally bonding with the child.

According to Buscaglia (1993), having a child with a malformation requires a tremendous emotional effort on the part of parents to give up fantasies of idealization. This process is slow and forces them to go through situations of denial, guilt, confusion, anger and despair. To better understand this process, we have developed some insights into parenting and its representations, the child's skills, and the parent-child relationship.

The purpose of this book is to review the topic of central nervous system malformations with emphasis on myelomeningocele. Analyze embryonic changes, clinical and surgical procedures, family relationships, socioeconomic status, quality of life and psychological aspects.

CHAPTER I.

EMBRYOGENESIS OF THE CENTRAL NERVOUS SYSTEM

Flavio Freinkel Rodriguez.
Mauricio Moscovici

The principles of body organization in vertebrates defined by the Genome are common: polarization, antimeria, metameria, stratimeria, and pachymeria. Let us emphasize two that are of particular interest for this paper: pachymeria and metameria. Pachymeria refers to the formation of two "tubes", a neural tube and a visceral tube. The dorsal tube, or neural pachymera, represents the central nervous system. The visceral pachymera corresponds to the thoracic and abdominal cavities.

The nervous system, located in the dorsal pachymere, is responsible for the relationship with the environment, given its origin from the ectoderm. Its cell outgrowths are distributed over the body surface, maintaining continuous communication with the environment, while in the soma it establishes posture and displacement and maintains visceral functional balance. Development occurs in parallel with organogenesis in the ventral pachymere and in the metameric organization of somites and their derivatives - sclerotomes. myotomes and dermatomes.

The process of nervous system development is the most complex in a living organism. In its completed form, the nervous system consists of approximately one million neurons and perhaps five to ten times that number of support and defense cells. Cells of the germ sheet differentiate and migrate under genomic control to form specialized structures. At least fifty thousand neurons are formed every second, they self-organize, and then most of them disappear as a result of cell death. The genome consists of approximately forty thousand genes.

The cell mass of the blastocyst consists of two primitive layers: ectoderm and entoderm. The embryo at this stage is a pear-shaped plate. With the appearance of notochordia at the edge of the neural canal, originating from the entoderm to the nerve plate

The primitive cells of the nerve plate, which form the proliferative layer, give rise to new concentric layers during mitosis. Undifferentiated cells of the germinal sheet are stem cells of the CS, which form the ependymal layer that covers the entire neural tube from the inside. New cells appear and differentiate into neuroblasts and spongioblasts. Neuroblasts give rise to neurons, while spongioblasts give rise to astrocytes and oligodendrocytes, which form the glia. Differentiation occurs in two phases. These cells proliferate rapidly and migrate centrifugally to form two layers: an inner layer next to the ependymaria, dominated by neuroblasts and neurons, called the mantle layer, and an outer layer composed of spongioblasts and their derivatives, astrocytes and oligodendrocytes. The mantle layer forms the gray matter and the marginal layer forms the white matter. Outgrowths of glial astrocytes cover the neural tube from inside and outside, acting as inner and outer boundary membranes. Neurons migrate along pathways spanned by astrocytes and controlled by genetic and functional factors. The displacement of neurons is called neurobiotaxis. Neuronal displacement and positioning is a complex process also activated by chemicals (SCHEIBEL, 2006).

The movements of neurons and astrocytes are also related to cellular structure: cells have a gelatinous surface on a less viscous endoplasm. This gelatinous lamina exerts a contractile tension, facilitating displacement (LEWIS, 1950).

During their movement, astrocytes form a dorsal cerebral septum along the dorsal part of the neural tube, in the marginal layer. This septum corresponds to the line of closure of the neural tube.

Myelomeningocele is a congenital malformation resulting from a neurulation disorder leading to exposure of a specific part of the spine.

Two theories have already been proposed to explain neural tube opening defects in myelomeningocele and anencephaly: the theory of nonclosure due to localized neurulation disorder and the theory of neural tube overstretching and rupture.

The theory of neural tube nonclosure due to impaired neurulation seems to be the most generally accepted mechanism, since neural tube closure depends primarily on the complex interaction of multiple cellular processes, the result of which may be a wide variety of processes. Embryologic lesions. Although there are many possible mechanisms, defects in neural tube opening and the causes of malformations in humans remain unknown (J. GORDON AND MCCOMB, 2008).

Midline fusion defect , also called cystic spinal cleft, resulting from insufficient primary neurulation. The term "dysraphism" or "fusion defect" as applied to the spine refers to injuries in which the neural tissue of the spinal cord is exposed to the environment and often accompanied by a liquor fistula. They are associated with malformations that affect the neural ectoderm between the leaflets that form the midline and skin, while laterally there is mesoderm that migrates between two folds of ectoderm to form the posterior arch of the vertebra (J. GORDON AND MCCOMB, 2008).

The process of secondary neurulation occurs when a mass of caudal cells migrate into the posterior neuropore, and it is a phenomenon that marks the end of primary neurulation. It forms a neurotubule through the process of canalization and fusion. It is a dysraphic disorder characterized by partial closure of the neural tube as a result of inadequate proliferation of ectodermal cells in the 3rd" 4th week of embryogenesis. (J. GORDON & MACCOMB, 2008).

Although neural tube closure defects have a heterogeneous etiology and several mechanisms of their occurrence have been described, most cases are due to the interaction of several genes and environmental factors, which is termed multifactorial inheritance. The mechanism of the genetic mechanism is not yet fully understood, but there is strong evidence for its involvement. Studies have shown that first line relatives have a higher risk of developing a neural tube closure defect than more distant relatives. Another evidence is the presence of neural tube closure defect in some genetic syndromes such as Meckel-Gruber syndrome, Waardenburg syndrome and trisomies of chromosomes 13 and 18 (MELVIN, 2000).

Several genes are thought to be involved in neural tube closure. Some of these genes may confer a strong genetic component, whereas others may have only a small effect when interacting with other genes. The most studied candidate genes are those related to folic acid metabolism, such as 5,10-methylenetetrahydrofolate reductase. Several investigators have reported a significant increase in the frequency of homozygotes for the C677T mutation of this gene in diseased individuals as well as in their mothers. (MELVIN, 2000).

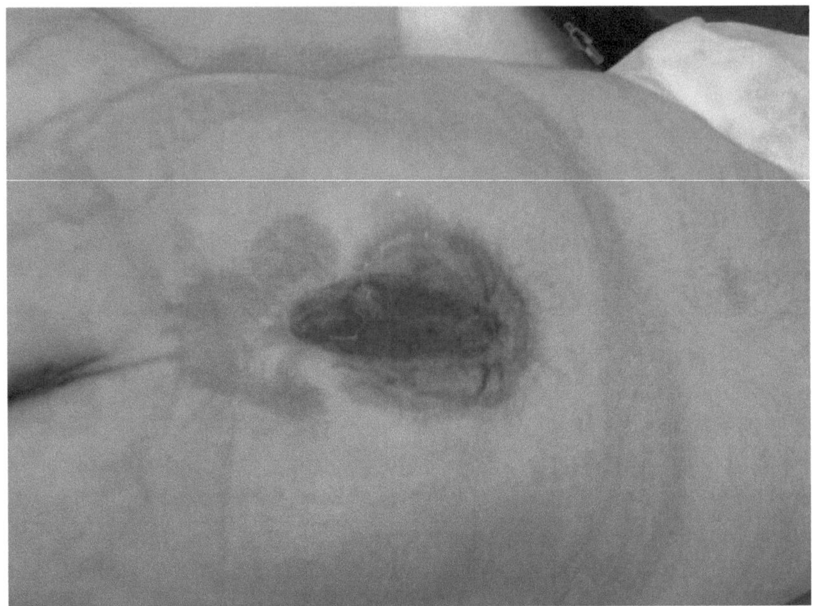

Source: Personal archive. Figure #1. Route of myelomeningocele (Personal archive)

In addition to genes, several environmental factors also appear to be involved in the etiology of neural tube closure defects. Folic acid is the most important risk factor identified to date. Other possible teratogenic agents are maternal diabetes mellitus, maternal use of valproic acid for epilepsy, maternal obesity, zinc deficiency and hyperthermia. (HARRIS, 1999).

Surgical repair

The anatomy of myelomeningocele can be visualized as concentric circles of normal tissue in abnormal locations. The innermost circle, or placode, consists of nerve elements that fuse under normal circumstances to form the neural tube and then the spinal cord. This central circle is usually fused with the surrounding epithelium. During surgical correction, the connections between the placode and the epithelium are delicately excised. The placode is mobilized, a tube is created, and it is secured with a thin thread, creating a surface , most of which is covered by the dura mater except for the area of the suture itself.

This pial surface is less likely to be attached to scar tissue. The next concentric circle of myelomeningocele is the dura mater. This tissue is usually mobilized from existing dysplastic bone elements. The dura mater is dissected free, sometimes reinforced with muscle and fascia, then brought to the midline and sutured tightly. Appropriate flaps of skin and fascia are brought to the midline and sutured. Sometimes it is necessary to close large defects with rotation of skin flaps and other soft tissues or with the use of relaxing incisions. Consultation with a plastic surgeon is appropriate in some situations. (FLANNERY AM 2010).

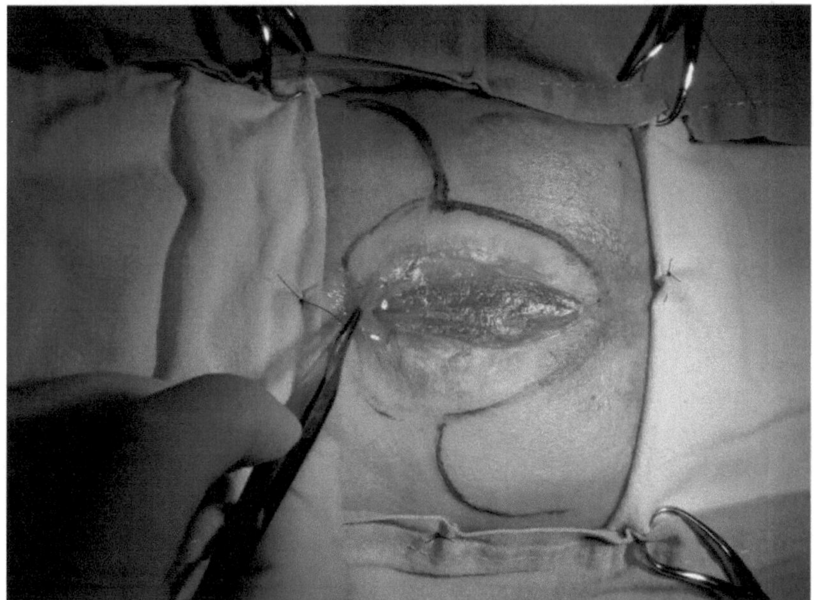

Source: Personal archive. Figure #2 Ruptured myelomeningocele. Surgical technique

Surgical treatment of myelomeningocele

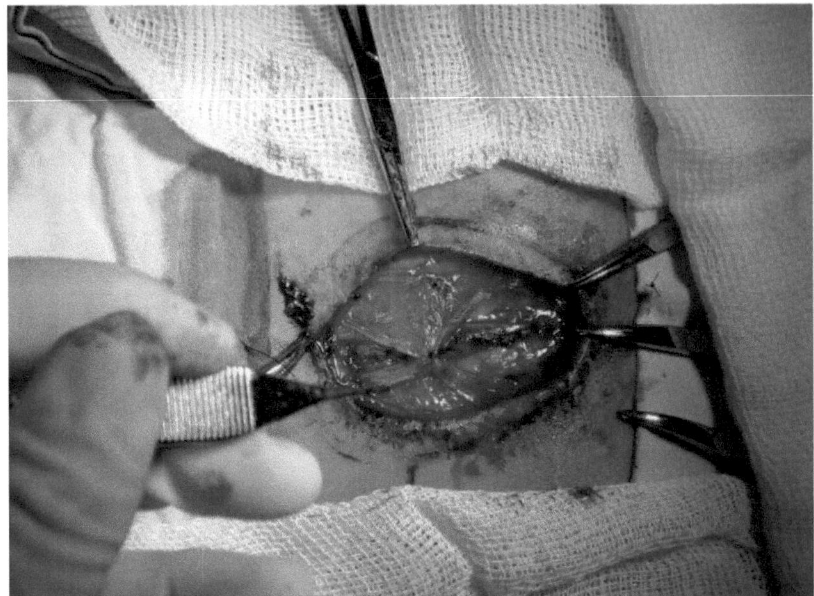

Source: Personal archive. Figure #3. Myelomeningocele. Surgical treatment.

Time to indication for surgery: it is generally accepted that early closure of a focal myelomeningocele may not result in improved neurologic function but prevents meningitis. Myelomeningocele injury should be repaired within 24-48 hours after birth. After approximately 36 hours, the lesion site begins to colonize with bacteria, and the incidence of postoperative infections tends to increase. Although the primary benefit of early closure of myelomeningocele is to reduce infection, it is also critical to preserve nerve tissue and blood supply.

Surgical Technique: The aim of the operation is to identify as many anatomical layers as possible and perform a watertight closure. In general, the following steps are performed:

1. Neural placode clearly separated from spider sheath, around membrane and ectodermal elements dissected. Preserved fragments

2. Skin tissue and epithelium that may cause a dermoid cyst must be removed.

3. The nerve tube is carefully reconstructed, and the placode is buried along the midline and sutured with nonabsorbable monofilament. Closure of the placode pia-pia may prevent reattachment of the terminal part of the spinal cord.
4. An examination of the end of the thread is made. This is separated if it is thickened.
5. In the dural sac, the dissection extends anteriorly into the spinal canal and laterally to the dermis. The most important step in the procedure is to determine the boundaries of the dura mater and dermis. In the dura mater, the incision is made circumferentially at the edge, separating it from the subcutaneous tissue and moving to the midline, where it is sutured.
6. Mesodermal elements such as muscles and fascia are displaced laterally; once the dura mater is closed, these layers are difficult to connect, but should be attempted if there is insufficient tissue.
7. Finally, the skin is mobilized by separating it from the lateral fascia and then tightening it to the midline. In large lesions or when the skin edges are under tension, a skin or musculocutaneous flap may be required to close the lesion postoperatively. After trauma recovery, it is important to keep the patient in a supine position to avoid pressure on the incision. A protective gown below the incision is used to prevent contamination with urine or feces. Head circumference is measured daily, and weekly head ultrasound is performed to evaluate for progressive ventriculomegaly, especially in children who do not have shunts.

Bladder procedure: catheterization to correct bladder function. Orthopedic care is important for future planning and correction of deformities of the limbs, hips or spine.

Other neural tube defects:

Chiari malformation II

It is a complex hindbrain anomaly detected by imaging studies. Only about 5 to 10 percent of people with symptomatic myelomeningocele are associated with Chiari II malformation. The malformation consists of a roof drop, organ torsion and elongation of the brainstem below the greater occipital foramen, and herniation of the cerebellar worm below the greater occipital foramen. The bony posterior fossa is usually small. Symptoms of this problem include difficulty breathing, cranial nerve palsy, especially palsy of nerves VI, VII, IX, and X, hypotonia, spasticity, and quadriparesis.

About 30 percent of children die from respiratory complications. Those people who have symptoms in childhood or adolescence usually do well. Magnetic resonance imaging (MRI) is the best test to detect Chiari II malformation. The severity of the disorder seen on imaging correlates poorly with the clinical presentation. Treatment usually includes laminectomy of the upper levels of the cervical spine and in some cases removal of the posterior margin of the greater occipital foramen to decompress the posterior fossa contents. The dura should be opened and a dural graft implanted. Some authors advocate dissection of the dura of the entire vermicular segment. Hydromyelia may occur. Hydromyelia often disappears after decompression of Chiari II malformation.

Meningocele

Much less common than myelomeningocele, meningocele is a variant of spinal cleft in which the cerebral membranes are stretched, often resulting in stretching or swelling of the skin and underlying tissues. The spinal cord and nerves are of normal configuration.

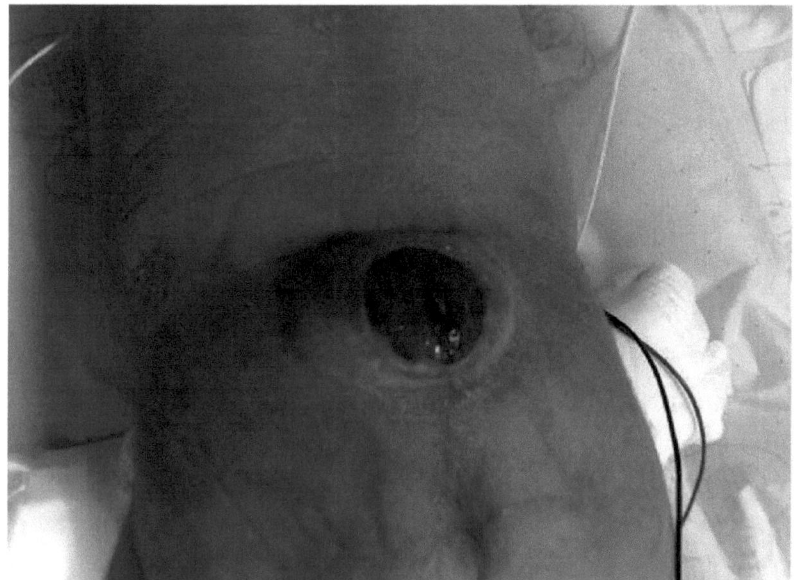

Source: Personal archive. Figure #4. Ruptured myelomeningocele in the lumbosacral region.

Spina bifida occulta or latent spinal dysraphism.

The embryology of myelomeningocele is well understood, but hidden spinal cleft is different and remains obscure. As in open spinal cleft, normal conditions and normal elements are present but in an abnormal location. The simplest form of concealed spinal cleft is probably filament thickening. More complex anomalies include lipomyelomeningocele anchored in the spinal cord and diastematomyelia.

Frame #1.

CLINICAL ADVICE<	**OCCULT spine development.**
SYSTEMS	**SIGNALS**
skin	Asymmetry of the gluteal fold, Capillary hemangioma, Hypertrichosis, Lipoma.

Neurological	Weakness in the lower extremities
Sensory deficit	Gait instability
Orthopedic	Low back and lower extremity pain, dropped foot, increased plantar arch, muscle atrophy, scoliosis
Urological	Incontinence

Source: ACOSTA and GUPTA, 2006.

Dermal sinus

Dermal sinuses extending from the epidermis to the deeper layers often penetrate through the dura mater into the subarachnoid space. Externally, the breast has the appearance of a pogo or dimple, often with a tuft of hair or opening along the midline. Cutaneous sinuses are most commonly found in the lumbosacral region, but may occur in conjunction with any midline structure, including the lower tip of the nose, occipital bone, and cervical spine.

Dermal sinus is often an asymptomatic malformation, but when it extends through the dura mater, it may be associated with recurrent meningitis. Therapy for dermal sinus and its resection.

Magnetic resonance imaging can help diagnose congenital malformations associated with anomalies that may include thickened filaments, fatty filaments, lipomas, or epidermoid tumors. The planned excision should be complete. The skin cavity should be traced along its entire length. This may include laminectomy and dissection of the dura mater, as well as surgical correction of associated soft tissues.

Fixed bone marrow

Although initially any lesion that fixes the spinal cord is often asymptomatic, it puts the individual at risk for possible neurologic dysfunction that may occur during periods of growth or during periods of adipose tissue deposition, which in addition to fixing neural structures may be associated with lipomatous lesions to increase the severity of malformation.

Signs and symptoms may be manifested by pain, in most cases the main clinical presentation is loss of bowel or bladder control, loss of sensation in the legs, or motor dysfunction in the sacral region and lower lumbar segments.

Surgical treatment of any injury causing spinal cord fixation is aimed at resecting the fixation. When the filum terminale thickens, there may be an associated lipoma.

The most elementary form of spinal cord fixation occurs when the filum terminale is excessively thick. In these cases, the filum terminale is often infiltrated with fatty tissue, as the filum is normally a fibrous structure. Resection of the spinal cord attachment is indicated when studies show that the conus is located below L2 in an adult or below L3 in a child. Surgical treatment of a thickened terminal filament includes laminectomy, opening of the dura mater, and dissection of the thickened filament. With early detection of terminal filament thickening, neurologic dysfunction can be prevented or, in some cases, reversed.

The embryologic development of bone marrow lipoma is still poorly understood. As in other forms of spinal anomalies, normal elements are present but in an abnormal position. One hypothesis is that these changes occur during the embryologic developmental phase after closure of the neural tube.

Treatment of entrenched bone marrow consists of resection of adipose tissue and release of bone marrow. Laminectomy, dissection of the dura mater and resection of lipomatous tissue and effective release of the spinal cord.

The surgical carbon dioxide laser is very useful in removing fatty tissue without damaging nerve structures. "The laser allows decompression and release without harming the spinal cord and nerve roots.

Lipomyelomeningocele

Lipomyelomeningocele is often found as fatty nodules on the back, usually in the lumbosacral region. Lipomyelomeningocele, which is often confused with an aesthetic deformity, is actually a complex congenital anomaly that manifests not only lipomatous elements and fatty infiltration in the neural tissues, as in lipoma, but also an associated meningocele or myelomeningocele. All of this abnormality can be covered by the skin.

Surgical correction of this condition includes removal of ligaments, lipomatous tissue, and reconstruction of the dural sheath of the spinal cord. As with all injuries in which spinal cord fixation compromises neurologic function, treatment should include reconstruction of these tissues before permanent damage occurs.

Diastematomyelia

A relatively rare manifestation of spinal dysraphism is diastematomyelia, a condition that includes the following components:

1. The spinal cord is divided, usually asymmetrically, into two hemimedullae. The dura mater may or may not be divided and surround each hemimedulla separately.
2. A protruding point on the vertebral body, consisting of bone or cartilage, may further separate the two semimedullae.
3. Diastematomyelia usually occurs in the thoracic or thoracolumbar region, and the vertebral body is associated with a malformation. Other congenital anomalies, such as semispinalis, are usually combined (FLANNERY, 2010).

BIBLIOGRAPHIC REFERENCES

1. ACOSTA F., GUPTA N. Spinal dysraphism. c.8:143-148, in Pediatric Neurosurgery, eds Frim D.M., Gupta I.N., eds Landes Bioscience. Georgetown, Texas, USA, 2006.

2. AGUIAR MJB, CAMPOS AS, AGUIAR RALP, LANA AMA: Neural tube defects and associated factors in liveborn and stillborn infants. Journal of Pediatrics (Rio de Janeiro) 79(2):129-34, 2003.

3. BERNARDES et al. Ultrasonographic diagnosis and neurologic prognosis in fetuses with myelomeningocele. Women's Gen; 34(12): 839-842, 2006.

4. BRAZIL, Ministry of Health. Information system on live births - SINASC. Brasilia: Ministry of Health; 2017.

5. MS DNI; McLONE DG cap. 21 pp.338-366 in Principles and Practice of Pediatric Neurosurgery. Albright, A.L.; Pollack, I.F. and Adelson, P.D., eds Thieme, 2nd ed. 2008.

6. FLANNERY A. M.: Diagnosis and surgical treatment of congenital lesions of the nervous system. Chapter 7 of Fundamentals of Neurosurgery, 7th [edition] , Tim, New York, 2010.

7. GORDON J. and MACCOMB. Spinal meningocele, Chapter 20, pp. 323-337 in Principles and Practice of Pediatric Neurosurgery. Albright, A.L., Pollack, I.F., and Adelson, P.D., eds. Scheibel, A.B. - Embryologic development of the human brain. 2006.

8. LEWIS, W.H. - Video imaging of neurons and neuroglia in tissue culture. In WEISS, P. - Genetic Neurology, University of Chicago Press, 1950.

9. HARRIS, M.J., JURILOFF, D.M.: Mini review: toward understanding the mechanism of genetic neural tube defects in mice. Teratology, 60, 292-305, 1999.

10. McLAWN, D.G.: Continuing concepts in the treatment of cleft spine. Pediatric Neurosurgery 18:254-256, 1992.

11. MELLO J. MHP, GOTTLIB SLD, SOBOL MLMS, ALMEIDA MF, LATORRE MRDO, Evaluation of a live birth information system and the use of its data in epidemiology and health statistics, SP1993, Ver. Saude Publica (6 supplements), 1993. .27

12. MELVIN S.E., GEORGE T.M., Worley G., FRANKLIM A., MACKIE J., WILES et al. Genetic studies of neural tube defects. Pediatr Neurosurg 2000; 32:1 -9

13. PERRY VL, OLBRIGHT AL, ADELSON PJ Operative nuances of myelomeningocele closure. Neurosurgery, 51(3):719-23, 2002.

14. Scheibel, A.B., Embryologic development of the human brain. Seattle, Washington. New horizons for learning. Retrieved February 2006 via the Internet: Neurobiology News:
    http//: www.newhorizons.org/neuro/scheib el.htm

15. ZAMBELLI H, MALDAUM MVC Cirurgia da Mielomeningocele 45: 501-504 in: A treatise on surgical technique in neurosurgery, ed. by Ateneu, São Paulo, 2009.

CHAPTER II

SOCIO-ECONOMIC ASPECTS OF CONGENITAL MALFORMATIONS

Eliete Botelho Cardoso

Family

Initially, the concern of the family in which a child with a malformation is born is centered on caring for the child, with doubts about survival, nutrition, and care. Later, there are concerns about structural deformity.

According to Santos (1995), family difficulties can interfere with a child's psychological development because growth and development depend on how they are perceived. Taking on the task of daily care of a child with a congenital deformity is not easy at first, and it becomes important for the family because they actually want to take responsibility for the care.

According to Gongalves, cited by Santos and Diaz (2005), the level of acceptance of a child with congenital anomalies will depend on the cultural background of the mother and the behavior of the family and may vary according to the social class to which he or she belongs.

The level of acceptance may be more prevalent among the financially less well-off classes, a result of cultural standards developed and internalized in terms of superstition and theological values, a resource that is widely used and resorted to religion, faith, to give meaning to the birth of a child with a malformation. In more privileged social classes, the difficulties of acceptance become greater as families are more aware of the obstacles, social stigma, the issues and pleasures they will be subjected to, and the difficulties of social integration of the child.

The acceptance of a new person into different social cultures must take place through "rituals of social transition," or more commonly called "rites of passage" (Hennep, 19, 78), even if they are not present in the minds of those who perform them. Ritual is a cultural system of symbolic communication. A study by Santos and Diaz (2005) revealed mothers' perceptions of children born with malformations related to conceptual references that discuss aspects of motherhood[1] and female sexuality from a psychoanalytic and cultural perspective, seeking to understand this meaning for women. Research has shown that social demands based on the figure of the "good mother" increase the insecurity of mothers of normal children in the role of "woman mother" and exacerbate feelings of failure in "women mothers of children." ugly children."

Pinheiro's study, cited by Santos and Diaz (2005), on the experiences of mothers with children with congenital malformations, presents an analysis of maternal reactions in order to characterize "being a mother" in their daily lives, seeking to understand this. phenomena, six units of meaning emerged:

- birth experience;
- Experience working with a child represented on therapeutic resources;
- hospital experience;
- Experience working with health care workers in a hospital setting
- experience in moments of distress.

According to Rubio (1999), through a qualitative study in the city of Rio de Janeiro of mothers' perceptions of prenatal and postnatal care for children with congenital anomalies, it showed that most mothers received care for nine months as normal pregnant women. three positions were identified in women, even if they presented high risk factors, regarding diagnostic information:

i According to Winnicott (2006, p. 30), pregnant women present a special mental state called primary maternal care. This state develops gradually and develops into a state of heightened sensitivity during and especially at the end of pregnancy, persisting for several weeks after the birth of the child.

- Full disclosure,
- Partial Information,
- Diagnosis omitted.

At discharge from the maternity hospital, most mothers were not informed about the disease, child care, were not warned about possible problems with the child, and sometimes they were not even referred to specialists and services to better address the characteristics of . problems (Rubio, 1999)

The events surrounding the birth of a child with special needs cause mothers to express feelings and actions about the situation that are often not understood by the professionals who help them.

Belli's study, cited by Santos and Diaz (2005), aimed to understand mothers' social representations regarding this situation. The study shows that the experience experienced by mothers is in fact a process of (re)signifying their social representations, this movement ensures the effective and legitimate participation of mothers with their child during hospitalization.

Most of the time the family, upon learning of the child's disfigurement, is gripped by panic, as if the child is being sentenced at that moment, as well as the family itself, not counting on this possibility, The family realizes that he is completely vulnerable in the face of the situation and can only define an intense fear of what he will have to face.

Research shows that when parents get the information and support they need, they tend to become more realistically accepting of the child. If there is no acceptance from a family member or the family as a whole, behavioral abnormalities can occur in this core. In the sense of not accepting or overprotecting the child (SANTOS, DIAS, 2005).

In the literature, we often find clear demonstrations of care for children with congenital malformations who require specialized attention and a multidisciplinary team, with a primary focus on maximizing recovery, including the child's integration into the family and social environment.

Knowledge of the issues of anatomy and physiology of treatment is not enough to support a more effective proposal of integrated care, it is necessary to know other factors that imply affective relationships between the child and his family members, family and social discrimination, because it is through the family that the child initially has access to the world (BUSCALIA, 1997).

We are individuals sharing our existence with like others, therefore we are individual and social beings, the first social group we belong to is the family and later we are gradually included in other social groups. Human beings need security and care from birth, the family and the social group initially responsible for these tasks are structured through roles and functions that determine the behavior that each person in that group will have.

In the core of the family we undergo transformations, as in any social environment, but the idea of family is a permanent axis of human nature, which is related to the regulation of kinship, procreation, sexual relations and the transmission of basic intermarriage. components of society aimed at actions aimed at the preservation and protection of the species, thus relational spaces emerge. The institution of the family is the first form of socialization created by human culture. In all societies, the idea of family relations represents a crystallized aspect in the mentality of individuals.

In general, through the family we are provided with a range of information that tells us who we are and what is expected of us socially. It is the basic unit of development where situations of achievement and failure, health and illness occur. It is a complex system of relationships within which there are interactions that do or do not contribute to the healthy development of its components (BUSCAGLIA, 1997).

In recent years, the family has been undergoing changes in its organizational structure, today it is common to see families run only by mothers or fathers from broken marriages, as well as families headed by single fathers or mothers, homosexuals, transgender persons, etc. the multiplicity of structures of family members, a reflection of a society that is trying to adapt to the accelerated pace of change. However, it can be observed that among this diversity of structures called family, the majority is a fairly stable organization in which the roles of each member are defined and rules of coexistence are established, indicating common values.

Buscaglia (1997, p. 84) states that:

" When these aspects of coexistence are harmonized, there is a reduction in problems, decision-making burdens, and the need for fundamental changes in family structure."

Another important observation to note is that although the family is a single group, it is situated in a broader social context, starting with the community as the first extension of the broader context, for example: the family, which is embedded in a broader context. the community, which consists of neighborhoods, schools, churches.... etc., which are also located in a neighborhood that belongs to a municipality, that belongs to a state, and that belongs to a nation.

Families in general are influenced by social determinants, and they also respond to this influence. "Values and customs adopted and disseminated within this wider social context will have a direct impact. A healthy family is a space of support, understanding and acceptance. Your organization provides an environment that guarantees the individuality and pursuit of fulfillment of its members. It serves as a safe training ground for experiences that will be meaningful for all its members" (BATISTA; FRANCA, 2007).

In essence, the role of the stable family is to offer a safe training ground where children can learn to be human, to love, to form their unique personality, to develop their self-esteem, and to interact with society at large. and changeable, out of what and for what they are born. (BUSCAGLIA, 1997).

Social consequences of malformations of the central nervous system

Lifestyle is increasingly becoming a risk factor for birth defects, as certain habits such as smoking, illicit drug use and alcoholism cause negative effects during pregnancy.

Other factors such as inadequate maternal nutrition, prenatal care, low level of education, self-medication, if associated with other factors, cause greater instability in the occurrence of congenital malformations.

Social factors are those that are not categorized as genetic components or physical, chemical or biological aggressors, including those that encompass socioeconomic, socio-political, sociocultural and psychosocial factors that allow a dialectical cognition of the patient and the disease itself, providing an understanding of the totality of reality (NAZER, LOPEZ, CASTILLA, 2001).

Other teratogenic agents that are possibly risk factors for birth defects are: maternal diabetes mellitus, use of valproic acid to treat epilepsy during pregnancy, maternal obesity, zinc deficiency, and hyperthermia (NAZER, LOPEZ, & CASTILLA, 2001).

Obesity is a factor that is on the rise worldwide and affects women of reproductive age, with numerous factors associated with weight gain, including infertility and pregnancy-related complications.

Many women of childbearing age resort to gastroplasty as a weight loss strategy, leading to an increase in the number of pregnant women undergoing this type of post-operative procedure. This surgical procedure can lead to serious nutritional complications, so there is speculation that this type of surgery can lead to an unfavorable pregnancy outcome for both mother and fetus. (JOSEPHSON, BLAD, VIREN, SIDSCHO, 2013).

It is very important to plan pregnancies in patients who have previously undergone gastroplasty with nutritional aspects in mind, as these patients may develop deficiencies in certain compounds such as iron, vitamin B12, folic acid and calcium, and this may lead to an increased risk of maternal complications. complications such as anemia, and fetal complications such as neural tube defect and intrauterine developmental delay (YOZEFSON, BLAD, VIREN, SIDSHO, 2013).

On this topic, there are still not enough studies giving us concrete scientific information on pregnancy outcomes after gastroplasty, with conflicting opinions arising mostly from clinical cases and studies with reduced casuistry. We cannot say with scientific certainty that poor nutrition in post-bariatric pregnant women is a favorable cause of fetal malformations, studies are still recent.

Thus, the factors that cause disease, whether biological or environmental, have complex social significance because society, while providing protection, determines the risks of disease. Varies according to greater or lesser access to measures to prevent disease and restore health (KNUPP, 2010).

According to the Organic Law on Social Assistance (LOAS), which defines persons with disabilities as "persons unable to work and lead an independent life," is completely contrary to the spirit of the global movement in favor of the social inclusion of these citizens and to the Federal Constitution itself. which, in line with this movement, contains several mechanisms aimed at improving living conditions and restoring citizenship. It also contradicts the global proposal for equal rights and health for all and the public health proposals for care provided to patients who seek to. reduce disability and promote autonomy.

Economic consequences of malformations of the central nervous system

The World Health Organization established the International Day of Persons with Disabilities to promote and deepen debate and knowledge on this topic and to mobilize support for the dignity, rights and well-being of people with special needs.

According to a 2006 publication by the Pan American Health Organization, only 2% of the 85 million people with disabilities have received adequate assistance in Latin America; the UN also warns that 80% of people with disabilities live in developing countries, in total, according to UNICEF, 150 million children (under 18) have a disability (PAHO, 2006).

According to WHO, as of 2011, 1 billion people are living with a disability, which means one in seven people in the world, the lack of statistics on persons with disabilities contributes to the invisibility of these people, which is an obstacle to planning and implementing development policies that improve the lives of people with disabilities, these citizens are often left without access to constitutionally acquired rights, the lack of ramps that provide better accessibility and inadequate health services are some of the examples that put p

Promoting and protecting the rights and dignity of people with disabilities is one of the important health and social well-being objectives addressed by PAHO. It emphasizes that there is a strong link between poverty and disability and that 80% of people with disabilities. live on low incomes.

Access to treatment and other health and educational services is limited by financial conditions, stigmatization of the disease, and exacerbated by prejudice and misinformation. Their ability to work may be limited by their physical disability and by lack of opportunity and prejudice on the part of employers. This set creates a vicious circle that needs to be broken.

In Brazil, the 1988 Federal Constitution (CF) grants specific rights to patients with disabilities, aimed at promoting their social integration. Although we have seen some progress, the situation is far from ideal (BRAZIL, 1988).

In the specific case of children born with MFC, research has shown that access to preventive and appropriate treatment and other basic essential services can change the stories of these individuals, helping to improve their self-esteem and enabling them to become physically, mentally and socially more independent. stigma, prejudice and lack of knowledge continue to be major barriers to this, especially when the population is most in need.

The proposed therapy requires follow-up with several specialists, often requiring hospitalization of the child for surgery and longer treatment, the family's lack of resources to pay for treatment often limits the possibility of seeking adequate medical care. which, because it is specialized, is rarely available in most basic health facilities, usually these specialties are concentrated in large service centers (ELIAS, MONTEIRO E CHAVES, 2008).

Thus a vicious circle is formed, since the lack of adequate and preventive treatment leads to more serious physical complications, increasing the need for better medical treatment, which consequently hinders the recovery of health and reduces the child's ability to attend school, as well as their own ability. to learn, leading to even greater isolation, damaging their social integration and their health in general (ELIAS, MONTEIRO E CHAVES, 2008).

Social rights aim to ensure that a person's daily and ongoing needs are met, ensuring equal opportunities such as the right to education, health, recreation and work. Access to these rights tends to be facilitated when people with disabilities and low family income start receiving the Continuation Payment Allowance (BPC), a free pass and enrollment in a school near their place of residence to increase family income. is demanded, but there are some difficulties in obtaining it.

As provided in Art. 203, V of the Federal Constitution and according to Brazil (2007):

Social assistance benefits will be provided to those who need them, regardless of Social Security contributions.

"Article 203. Social assistance will be provided to those who need it, regardless

of social security contributions, and its objectives are:

V - guarantee of a monthly benefit equal to the minimum wage for disabled and elderly persons who prove that they do not have the means to provide for their own maintenance or that of his family, as provided by law."

This benefit is governed by Law 8742/93, known as the Organic Law on Social Assistance (LOAS), and Decree 1744/95, which establish the following requirements for granting:

a) Be disabled or at least sixty-five (65) years of age for seniors who are not disabled;

b) Monthly family income (per capita) less than % of minimum wage;

c) Not to be associated with any social security scheme;

d) Receive no benefits other than medical care;

e) Prove that you do not have the means for your own maintenance or that your family is providing it;

To analyze the eligibility for the continuous social assistance benefit (BPC-LOAS) established by Law 8,742/93, the following will be considered:

a) Senior Citizens: persons sixty-five (65) years of age or older;

b) Person with a disability (PPD): is one who is incapable of independent living and working, that is, one who has a loss or diminution of his or her structure or anatomical, physiological, psychological or mental functions of a permanent nature due to abnormalities. or irreversible injuries of hereditary, congenital or acquired nature which result in an inability to live independently or to carry out activities within the limits considered normal for a person, as set out in National Classification 29 summary.

c) Disability: a multidimensional phenomenon that includes a limitation of activity and participation with an effective and marked reduction in the capacity for social inclusion, which corresponds to the interaction between the person with a disability and his or her physical and social environment;

d) Family: a group of people living under the same roof, including spouse, partner, parents, children, brothers and sisters, not exempted from any condition, under the age of twenty-one (21) years or disabled, as well as those treated as children, in the case of stepchildren and minors under guardianship (according to Article 16 of Law 8,213/1991);

e) Family unable to provide maintenance for a disabled or elderly person: a family whose per capita income calculation corresponds to the sum of the gross monthly income of all its members divided by the total number of members constituting the family group. The family's per capita income is less than 1/4 (quarter) of the minimum wage.

f) family for the calculation of the average per capita income provided for in Art. 20 para. Article 20(1) of Law 8,742/1993: a group of people living under the same roof, i.e. the applicant, spouse, partner, unemancipated child of any condition, under 21 years of age or disabled, parents and incapacitated children. -emancipated sibling of any condition, under 21 years of age or disabled;

Note[1] : A stepchild and a minor ward are equal to a child when there is proof of economic dependence and as long as they do not have sufficient assets for their own maintenance and education;

Note[2] : The son or brother of a disabled claimant who is not receiving Social Security or permanent benefits because of a disability or impairment must undergo an expert medical evaluation to confirm the disability.

g) Gross monthly family income: the sum of the gross income received monthly by family members, consisting of wages, earnings, pensions, alimony, public or private pension benefits, commissions, labor support contributions, other income from self-employment, market income, informal or self-employed. -workers, income derived from property, lifetime monthly income and permanent benefits allowance, except as provided for in the single paragraph of Article 19 of Decree 6,214/2007 (BRAZIL, 2007).

Although the applicant submits all necessary documentation and meets the required legal criteria, INSS may issue an opinion on the socio-economic status of the beneficiary's family, which may make it difficult or even prevent its receipt. It is important to emphasize that the World Bank classifies people with a per capita income of up to US$2 per day as poor and people with a per capita income of up to US$1 per day as extremely poor. Thus, the expected values of benefit receipt (% of minimum wage) are close to the extreme poverty line.

Article 1: Social assistance, a right of the citizen and an obligation of the State, is a non-contributory social security policy that provides a social minimum, realized through an integrated set of actions of public initiative and society, to guarantee the service. basic needs.

To analyze the entitlement to the continuous social assistance benefit (BPC-LOAS) established by Law No. 8742/93 will be considered as:

Disabled Person (IPD): is one who is incapable of independent living and working, that is, one who has a loss or reduction in his or her structure or anatomical, physiological, psychological or mental functions of a permanent nature, due to abnormalities or irreversible injuries of hereditary, congenital or acquired nature, resulting in an inability to live independently or to perform activities within the limits considered normal for a human being as defined in the JEF National Unification Class 29 summary;

Disability: a multidimensional phenomenon that includes a limitation of activity and participation with an effective and marked reduction in the capacity for social inclusion, which corresponds to the interaction between the person with a disability and his or her physical and social environment;

Family: a group of people living under the same roof, including spouse, partner, parents, children, brothers and sisters, not exempt from any condition, under the age of twenty-one (21) years or disabled, as well as those treated as children, in the case of stepchildren and minors under guardianship (according to Article 16 of Law No. 8213/1991);

Family unable to provide maintenance for a disabled or elderly person: a family whose per capita income calculation corresponds to the sum of the gross monthly income of all its members divided by the total number of members constituting the family group. A family whose per capita income calculation corresponds to the sum of the gross monthly income of all its members divided by the total number of members of the family group.

Family for the calculation of the average per capita income provided for in par. Article 20, paragraph 1 of Law No. 8,742/1993: a group of people living under the same roof, i.e. the applicant, spouse, partner, unemancipated child of any condition, under 21 years of age or disabled, parents and unemancipated brother or sister of any condition, under 21 years of age or disabled;

Gross monthly family income: sum of gross income received monthly by family members, consisting of wages, earnings, pensions, alimony, public or private pension benefits, commissions, labor support funds, other income from self-employment, income from informal or independent activities. -employment market, income derived from assets, lifetime monthly income and allowance with permanent payments, subject to the provisions of the single paragraph of Article 19 of Decree 6,214/2007 (BRAZIL, 2007).

Law No. 1941 guarantees free intercity travel (PIL) to people with chronic illnesses and persons with disabilities who have recognized mobility difficulties, on public passenger transport (road, metro, suburban and maritime) and who are enrolled in the public school closest to their place of residence.

Social integration

The social inclusion of people with disabilities has received more attention with the advent of the Brazilian Constitution of 1988, which recognizes that all people who make up society are equal and are citizens with responsibilities and rights.

Social inclusion is a process of positive attitudes, public and private, to include all those groups or populations that have been marginalized historically or as a result of current radical political, economic or technological changes into the broader social context. One aspect of the process of social inclusion is school inclusion, which is a set of public and private measures aimed at making schooling available to all segments of society, with a focus on childhood and youth.

In this context, the inclusion of people with special needs in mainstream schools is emphasized, education should focus on vocational training and awareness-raising for citizens.

The issue of people with disabilities has gained prominence in society as it is seen as a human rights issue. This achievement has occurred thanks to the mobilization of people with disabilities in search of their rights and by the United Nations (UN) this year. In this sense, the Convention on the Rights of Persons with Disabilities (CRPD), created by the UN in 2007, represents a milestone in the recognition of human rights, providing civil, cultural, political, social and economic rights to all without discrimination. The CRPD aims to "promote, protect and ensure the full and fair enjoyment of all human rights and fundamental freedoms by all persons with disabilities, and to promote respect for their inherent dignity." (BRAZIL, 2007).

We can observe that the legislation is in many cases poorly enforced by public authorities established in all spheres, most families do not find adequate treatment for their disabled child in any health center to provide treatment for the child, these families are constantly moving between different health centers, so they do not find uniformity in care, assistance and information.

BIBLIOGRAPHIC REFERENCES

BATISTA SM; FRANCA RM, The family of people with disabilities. Challenges and their overcoming. ICPGVol. scientific and technical journal. 3 н. January-June 10, pp. 117/2007ISSN18072836. http://www.ebah.com.br/content/ABAAABPiYAG/familia-pessoas-com-deficiencias-desafios-superacao .

BRAZIL. **Decree no. No. 6214 of September 26, 2007,** regulates the benefits for the continuation of social assistance to disabled and elderly people referred to in Law No. 8742 of December 7, 1993 and Law No. 10741 of October 1, 2003, adds a paragraph. to art. 162 of Decree no. 3048 of May 6, 1999 and other provisions. Available at: < https://www.planalto.gov.br/ccivil 03/Ato2007-2010/2007/Decreto/D6214.htm > . Accessed: 10 September 2018 BRAZIL.

BRAZIL, Constitution of the Federative Republic of Brazil, 1988, Title II, Fundamental Rights and Guarantees, Chapter I, Individual and Collective Rights and Duties, Article 1, Paragraph III, Chapter II, Social Rights, Article 5, Article 6 Constitutional Amendment No. 64. 2010, Article 23, Chapter II, Article 196, available at: http://www.planalto.gov.br/ccivil 03/constituicao/constituicao.htm , as of August 15, 2018.

BUSCALIA, L. Persons with disabilities and their parents. 3rd ed. Rio de Janeiro: Record, 1997. pp. 78 epub. 84.

Hennep, A.V. Rites of initiation. Petropolis: Voices, 1978. 181c.

VMAO KNUPP, Risk factors associated with neonatal mortality among a cohort of live births in the city of Rio de Janeiro in 2005. 2010. 122 f, p.19. Dissertation (Master of Nursing) - Alfredo Pinto School of Nursing, Federal University of the State of Rio de Janeiro (UNIRIO), Rio de Janeiro.

JOSEFSSON A, BLAD M, VIREN AB, SIDSHO G. **Risk of congenital malformations in offspring of women who have undergone bariatric surgery** . A national cohort. BJOG. 2013;120(12):1477-82. doi: 10.1111/1471-0528.12365.

ORGANIC SOCIAL ASSISTANCE LAW (LOAS), Benefit for the Continuous Provision of Social Assistance-BPC-LOAS for the Elderly and People with Disabilities http://www.previdencia.gov.br/conteudoDinamico.php?id=23/http://www.planalto.go v.br/ccivil_03/leis/l8742.htm. Accessed July 20, 2018.

NAZER JD, LOPEZ CARMELO JC, CASTILLA EE ECLAMC: A 30-year epidemiologic surveillance study of neural tube defects in Chile and Latin America. Rev Med Chil 2001;129:531.

OPAS. Pan American Health Organization. Resolution CD47.R1 "Disability: Prevention and Rehabilitation in the Context of the Right to the Highest Possible Standard of Physical and Mental Health and Other Related Rights", September 2006.

RUBIO SA. Reports of mothers of children with congenital anomalies on the care received during pregnancy: a comparative study in Rio de Janeiro/Brazil and Piura/Peru [dissertation]. p.21 Rio de Janeiro (RJ): Anna Neri School of Nursing, Federal University of Rio de Janeiro; 1999.

SANTOS MS. Being a mother of a special child: from dream to reality [abstract]. Rio de Janeiro (RJ): Anna Neri School of Nursing, Federal University of Rio de Janeiro; 1995. p.05

SANTOS RS; IMV DAYS. Reflections on birth defects. Rev. bras. enferm. p.04, vol. 58#5, Brasilia, September/October 2005. http://dx.doi.org/10.1590/S0034-71672005000500017

WINNICOTT, D.V. Human Nature. Rio de Janeiro: Imago. 1990. 222c.

CHAPTER III

PSYCHOLOGICAL ASPECTS OF CONGENITAL MALFORMATIONS

Joanna Ayla Donzelli Schultz.

Considerations about parenting: parents' perceptions

The term "parenthood" appeared in French literature in the 1960s to refer to the process of becoming a mother and father. The term denotes the scale of the process and the construction of the bond between parents and children (ZORNIG, 2010).
According to some authors (Stern, 1997; Zornig, 2010; Lebovici, 1987), parenthood is not limited to pregnancy and childbirth, as the personal history of the parents will influence and determine the establishment of emotional bonds with the child. . child.
According to Seyer, "the prehistory of the child is linked to the history of the man, the woman, and the couple they form, from their meeting to their common project or lack of pregnancy" (2002, p. 188).
The process of becoming a mother and father begins in the childhood of parents, through the identification they have with their parents and ancestors, and continues, lasting a lifetime and triggering a wide variety of desires and feelings.
The desire to have a child is a complex process generated by the diverse experiences and fantasies present in the history of parents. It can renew childhood fantasies as well as the forms of care that each parent received from their parents. The birth of a child depends on the desire of each spouse as well as their own desire for life. The desire may be unconscious or conscious, but it must be present for conception to occur and pregnancy to take place. (ZORNIG, 2010).
According to Brazelton and Kramer (1992), identification, the desire for completeness and duplicity, the desire to reflect oneself in the child, and the desire to realize ideas and possibilities lost to parents are just some of the fantasies present in the process of becoming children. becoming a mother and becoming a father.

The child's parents or caregivers will imitate their parents or caregivers and reproduce that care in childhood play. Years later, these identifications will influence the care given to the child by his or her parents.
The desire for fullness, as well as the desire to reflect oneself in the child, the authors

also refer to as the narcissistic needs of parents; deserving more attention when the child is born with a congenital malformation.

The term "narcissism" as used by Brazelton and Kramer (1992) refers to the mental work of "developing and maintaining an image of the self and the degree of investment in that very image" (p. 15).

According to the authors:

"A woman's cherished desire to bear a child contains within it the hope of self-reproduction. This hope supports the idea of immortality: the child will be a living testimony to the mother's continued existence. This desire for mirroring also embraces family ideals and traditions: the child represents the promise of continuity, the embodiment of these values. The child is seen as the next link in a long chain that connects each parent to his or her parents and ancestors" (BRASELTON & KREMER, 1992, p. 15).

Confirmation of pregnancy awakens new feelings in parents, including: euphoria of the first moment, awareness of future responsibilities, the desire to overcome their own capabilities, expectations about the child, and the fear of having a malformed child. The authors further state that "to overcome these fears and the underlying ambivalence, the mother-to-be needs to mobilize defenses and more defenses. You need to begin to idealize the child, seeing it as a perfect and fully loved being" (BRASELTON; KREMER, 1992, p.24). Thus, the possibility of having an ugly child is denied because it threatens the parents' self-esteem.

According to Lebovici (1987), there are three types of parental perceptions of the child: the phantom child, the imaginary child, and the real child. The phantom child is the child that is present in the parents' minds from childhood, it is unconscious and influences how the parents will care for the real child. The imaginary child is the one that is present in the couple's mind as a project, as it appears after meeting the parents and wanting children. This is the baby of the couple's dreams and expectations during pregnancy. The real baby is the one in the arms of their parents and may be similar to or very different from the imagined baby. There may be feelings of longing and ambivalent behavior toward the baby. Yet, according to Lebovici (1987), the initial ambivalence of mothers can be better understood by considering that the imaginary baby and the real baby are different, that is, one does not correspond to the other. Therefore, in addition to losing the imaginary child, parents will have to adjust to the demands of the real child.

Pregnancy and the postpartum period are described by some authors (Maldonado, 1997; Bydlowsky, 2002) as a crisis situation that requires parents to define a new role and adapt to the psychological and biochemical changes that occur during this period. Bydlowsky (2002) introduced the term *"psychic transparency"* to refer to a special state of the female psyche during pregnancy "in which fragments of the preconscious and unconscious easily reach consciousness" (2002, p.205). Pregnancy is understood by the author as a period of the crisis of adulthood experienced by a pregnant woman, which mobilizes her psychic energy, awakens anxieties and conflicts, but at the same time expands her potential and makes possible an intimate reunion of the pregnant woman with herself. Mental transparency, in the words of the author, "reactivates the child that the mother was or believed herself to be, which until then had remained hidden deep in her psyche" (2002, p.218).

Psychological changes during pregnancy and the postpartum period are experienced not only by women but also by men. According to Seyer (1999), parents also experience a number of transformations with the birth of their child. Some suffer from fractures and sprains a few days before birth, that is, they express their pain and insecurity with their bodies. Others experience similar symptoms during their wife's pregnancy, such as vomiting episodes, weight gain, and insomnia.

According to a study entitled "Father involvement during pregnancy" (PICCININI *et al.,* 2004), some fathers may also experience anxiety about childbirth, the health of the baby, the health of the mother, and a tendency toward Couvade behavior . Couvade syndrome is a set of symptoms that men may experience during pregnancy. They experience sensations similar to those of their pregnant partner, such as nausea, food cravings and bouts of crying.

According to Zornig (2010, p.458):

"Perceptions influence the different types of interactions that occur between a child and his or her caregivers, which can facilitate or hinder the establishment of safe emotional bonds."

Parenting role considerations

Although the influence of parent-child interactions on child development is not the focus of this paper, we consider this topic important because they are interrelated. Therefore, in this chapter we will briefly introduce parental roles and their possible influence on child development. Winnicott (1978) conducts an in-depth study of the mother's role in the earliest stages of child development and develops a concept he calls *primary maternal concern.* This is a very special psychological state experienced by the mother during pregnancy and immediately after the birth of the child. This state, according to the author, develops gradually and develops into a state of heightened sensitivity during and especially late in pregnancy. It continues for several weeks after birth and is not easily recalled when the mother has recovered. It is the opinion of this author that the mother's memory of this condition tends to be suppressed.

Primary maternal care allows the mother to adapt sensitively and sensitively to the initial needs of the child. The mother in this state creates the *conditions in* which the child's constitution can manifest itself, the child's developmental tendencies can begin to emerge, and the child can exhibit spontaneous movements. In this context, the child's own lifeline is hardly disturbed by reactions to intrusion. In the author's view, reactions to intrusion interrupt the child's "continued existence" and jeopardize the child's development. Overreaction does not cause frustration, but rather the threat of annihilation (WINNICOTT, 1978).

The mother's investment in the child contributes to the lake by strengthening the relationship between them, making the child capable of a personal existence. This relationship often begins intrauterine, as the fetus is able to hear and feel the sound of the mother's voice and mood.

Yet, according to Winnicott, a reasonably good mother performs three functions: holding, b) handling, and c) presenting objects . The term "holding" in the strict sense refers to the mother's ability to provide good "support" for the child; more specifically, it refers to the act of holding the child on her lap. In its broadest sense, it refers to the mother's ability to support, provide, provide what is necessary for the child's psychobiological survival.

According to Crespin (2004), the child is already a relational being before birth.

Birth also corresponds to a time of encounter. The author quoted above, speaking of this time, uses the expression *"primordial recognition".* It is an act of pure projection. Parents and family members identify themselves with the newborn, discovering physical and even behavioral similarities, thus integrating it into the family.

From this point on, parents can bring maternal and paternal functions into play. These functions are present in parents in unequal and variable forms, and sometimes in an inverted form (CRESPIN, 2004).

In order to get in touch with her baby, the mother takes herself for him, or rather, she takes him as part of herself. After birth, the mother continues to occupy an attributive place at the moment the exchange begins. In other words, the mother thinks about her baby and attributes mental content to it. She knows for her child as much as she knows for herself. (...) Men have a first child and a second child. (...) The child is not thought of as part of the self. The paternal function is the mental operator of separation. The paternal function corresponds to the father's separative capacity and his regulatory function to the mother's original omnipotence. (CRESPEN, 2004, p. 29)

But initially, the father also plays the role of supporting the mother/child dyad so that the mother can fulfill her role safely and securely. Support in this context means creating a supportive environment so that the mother can devote herself exclusively to the needs of the child. And if these are properly attended to, the child will develop physically and mentally so that he can build his subjectivity.

Initially, the child is born extremely dependent on care and the maternal function accepts this dependence, but for the mother-child relationship to be satisfactory, the mother must show herself capable of accepting the otherness of the child. The mother cannot decide everything for her child; she should not. The coldness she feels will not necessarily be felt by her child. For the child's psyche to develop, the mother must realize that she and her child are different beings with different desires . Through the paternal function, the child leaves its status as part of the mother and is no longer so predictable, completely understandable, completely at her mercy. The paternal function brings a dimension of otherness and thus guarantees space for the development of the child's psyche (CRESPIN, 2004).

Regarding the role of the father, Brazelton and Kramer state: "Recognizing the father's role not only assists the expectant mother in her task of separating herself from the fetus and differentiating him from her fantasies, but also reassures her that she is not only responsible for possible successes or failures" (1992, p.28).

Considerations on parent-child interactions in central nervous system malformations

Parents with their desires and life stories are not the only actors in the process of constructing parenthood, the child also plays an active and important role in establishing emotional connections with their parents.

Newborn skills

The primary need of the newborn is the need to be loved. Not just to be loved; but to be able to love. Ashley Montague

There is consensus among some authors (Lebovici, 1987, Bowlby, 1989, Ainsworth, 1989, cited by De Andrade, 2002) that parents' perceptions of the child and of themselves as parents influence parenting.

But if, on the one hand, parental representations are able to influence the relationship established between parents and child, on the other hand, contemporary studies reviewed by some authors, including Lebovici (1987), Bowlby (1989) and Claus and Kennell, (1992) show that the child is also actively involved in the process of parental formation and at birth possesses a number of characteristics that allow him/her to interact with his/her parents and caregivers . Thus, it can be stated that the concept of interaction acquires a new dimension by introducing the idea of reciprocity in the parent-child relationship.

According to Gols (2002), over the past four decades, their caregivers and early childhood researchers have begun to look at infants through different eyes. Before World War II, the infant was considered a passive being who spent most of his time eating, crying, and sleeping. In France, it was called an infant, clearly alluding to the central aspect of nutrition in its care. After the war, the infant came to be called a baby and:

"It has become synonymous with a much more active being, not only capable of eating, drinking, defecating, but also capable of immediate relations with others (...)" (GOLSE, 2002, p.117).

Brazelton and Kramer (1992) describe very well the feelings of the newborn that seem to contribute to the establishment of first bonds, viz:

- Vision: newborns prefer human faces and are able to fixate and follow the faces of their parents in the delivery room immediately after birth.
- The sense of hearing: some studies show that newborns are more interested in female voices and are calmer when they hear sounds that are in the sound frequency range of 500 to 900 vibrations per second, which is the range of human speech (EISENBERG, 1976, cited by BRASELTON & CREMER, 1992).
- Olfaction: in 80% of cases, infants at one week of age are able to distinguish their mother's funnel odor from that of other mothers (MACFARLANE, 1975, cited by BRAZELTON and CRAMER, p. 1992).
- Touch: touch represents an important means of communication between parent and child: "(...) it is a code shared by caregiver and child - both to soothe the child and to wake him or her up or warn him or her." (BRASELTON & KREMER, p. 74, 1992).

According to Stern (1992), infants interact with their parents from birth. The infant's main task is to establish contact with others. Through sights and sounds, the infant can request or refuse contact with its parents or caregiver. Parents, in turn, try to adjust to the baby's requests and needs. The development of attachment and emotional bonds between parents and children depends on this exchange of stimuli and mutual adaptation between the parties involved.

According to Brazelton and Kramer:

"(...) immediately after birth, babies synchronize their movements according to the rhythm of their mother's voice. Here is an example of the great power of mutual adaptation in early childhood. The baby's movements match the movements of the mother, who in turn adapts her speech to the baby's movements. Parents discover a pitch and rhythm of sound that captivates their child, who begins a kind of dance to the sound of the parents' voice" (1992, p.71).

Bowlby (1989), influenced by ethology, developed attachment theory, in which he believes that the establishment of emotional bonds between child and adults is aimed at guaranteeing the preservation of the species.

Attachment is a type of bond in which one's sense of security is closely tied to the object of attachment. In a relationship with an attachment figure, the security and comfort experienced in their presence allows the figure to be used as a "secure base" from which to explore the rest of the world (Bowlby, 1979/1997, cited by Ramirez & Schneider, 2010.)).

Based on Bowlby's (1989) concept of attachment, Ainsworth (1989), cited by De Andrade (2002) in an experiment called "The Strange Situation", described four attachment patterns, viz:

a) Secure attachment: A baby who develops this attachment pattern appears confident toward his parents and is sure that help will come in unfavorable situations. Parents respond immediately to the baby's calls, kindly and coherently.

b) Resistant and anxious attachment. In unfavorable situations, the baby is unsure of the availability and ability to get help or response from their parents. They react with separation anxiety and seek to be as close to their primary caregiver as possible.

c) Anxious attachment with avoidance: it is as if the baby does not expect help from parents in unfavorable situations, on the contrary, the baby expects to be rejected.

d) Disorganized attachment: the child develops apathy in the face of adverse experiences. Stop asking for help.

Research shows that when children are born with malformations, the process of adaptation of the parents to the child's needs and the new situation is more intense and full of suffering, and the parents go through a process similar to that of grieving. (BRASELTON and KREMER, 1992; GOMEZ, 2007; LEBOVICI, 1987; CLAUS and PITOMNICK, 1993).

The term congenital malformation (CM) refers to any functional or structural abnormality in fetal development resulting from a factor occurring before birth, genetic, environmental or unknown, even if the defect is not apparent in the newborn and only manifests itself later. (BELFORT, BRAGA, FREIR, 2006). In Brazil, VM is the second cause of infant mortality, accounting for 11.2% of all neonatal deaths (AMORIM *et al.,* 2006).

The government has taken some measures to reduce the incidence of DFTN and anemia, such as the approval of RDK Resolution No. 344 of December 13, 2002, which obliges the food industry to add for every 100 g of wheat flour, corn flour and cake mix, 150 µg of folic acid and 4.2 mg of iron (BRAZIL, 2002).

According to the Ministry of Health, folic acid supplementation should be taken prophylactically, in the pre-pregnancy period (12 weeks before pregnancy) and in the first three months of pregnancy, especially for women with a history of malformations, at a dosage of 5 mg/day (BRAZIL 2006). Some studies conducted in the United

States have confirmed the effectiveness of supplementing the diet of pregnant women with folic acid and showed a reduction of up to 70% of NTDF cases. (AMORIM et al., 2012).

Level of injury, orthopedic changes, family motivation, balance deficits, cognitive changes, and the presence of Arnold-Chiari type II malformation are among the factors considered important in establishing prognosis. Motor and sensory changes vary depending on the level of injury and degree of spinal cord injury (SOUZA et. al., 2007).

These children require intensive and continuous care throughout their lives as they may have serious disorders such as: hydrocephalus, neurogenic bladder, bowel dysfunction, orthopedic problems, lower limb paralysis and bone and joint anomalies (GAIVA and MODES, 2008). They are usually cared for by multidisciplinary teams in the fields of pediatrics, neurology, urology, orthopedics, psychology, speech therapy, physical therapy, occupational therapy and others depending on the severity of the illness and their needs. They also undergo a number of medical examinations and procedures, especially if they have more than one type of birth defects.

Impact of prenatal diagnosis and the birth of a child with a congenital malformation.

Prenatal diagnosis (PND) allows to monitor the development of the fetus and to detect some congenital anomalies before birth. The diagnostic methods used may vary for each pregnancy and are categorized as invasive (amniocentesis, blood tests) and non-invasive (ultrasound, Doppler) (SUASSUNA, 2010). DPN often provides early intervention and management of some malformations.

As mentioned earlier, over a long period of time, parents construct an image of their child according to their own identifications, aspirations and frustrations. And the birth of this child, even in a normal context, can cause parents to feel a sense of loss.

The grief experienced mainly by the mother concerns her new position, such as giving up her position solely as a daughter to become a mother, or even giving her autonomy to care for a being that depends on her (SZEJER, 2002).

The confrontation between the imaginary child and the real child can also arouse in parents a sense of loss, since the former never corresponds to the latter, and conflicts may arise interfering with the mother-child relationship (LEBOVICI, 1992).

Thus, the diagnosis of a child with a malformation can be seen as another crisis that exacerbates the losses suffered by the parents. The news that something is going wrong brings much distress to the couple and their families (MOREIRA et al. , 2006).

According to Moreira:

"When "something else" is detected in the fetus, the couple becomes uncomfortable. This 'something else' is usually an image detected during an ultrasound . Imaging technology has allowed the couple to get closer to their baby while still in utero. The ability to perceive details in the formation of a new being is useful in prenatal care, but can turn into anguish when changes occur that could pose a danger to the fetus. These include malformations, perinatal hemolytic diseases and threats of preterm birth" (2006, p. 16).

According to Suasuna:

"It must be emphasized that the speed of the encounter between Mother and Fetus through the on-screen image and the fact that the image communicates all elements at once only makes it more difficult for parents to prepare for this moment; hence the intensity, disorganization, and traumatic experience that can occur" (2010, p. 141).

Suassuna also warns that the impact of the news depends on: "structure, past history, needs, conflicts, the moment of current life, the relationship with the family, the place intended for the child, and the mother's ability to develop her mental representations. fetus (...) (2010, p.142)".

DPN for congenital malformations favors surgical intervention in the first 48 hours after birth and reduces the risk of complications in the child. The diagnosis is accurate and correct in most cases. On the other hand, the prognosis is uncertain and varies depending on the localization and severity of the malformation in the child.

Psychological reactions of parents and parent-child interactions with congenital malformation.

According to Lebovici (1987), the birth of a child with malformations usually causes great anxiety to the parents. The mother feels responsible and guilty for the abnormality of her child because she feels that she is producing an "imperfect" and "inferior" being. The malformation is not seen by the parents as a disease or symptom that can disappear, but rather as an abnormality that will accompany the child throughout life. Longing, helplessness and sadness take over the parent-baby relationship.

Brazelton and Kramer (1992) argue that having a child with a malformation leads to a drop in the mother's self-esteem and self-worth, the child is perceived as a result of maternal failure, and the bonding process may be harmed.

Some authors (Canavarro and Fonseca, 2010) argue that parents' initial reactions immediately after a diagnosis that something is going wrong are similar to grief reactions (shock, sadness, anxiety, guilt, and anger).

Klaus and Kennel (1993) identified the following phases in the organization of these reactions:

I - Shocker;

II - Denial;

III - Sadness and anger;

IV - Balance;

V - Reorganization.

Initially, immediately after receiving the news of the birth of a child with a malformation, couples are in a state of shock, emotionally "paralyzed". They tend to feel unprepared to cope with the situation and believe they will not be able to survive it, and exhibit running away, crying fits and lack of emotional control.

In the denial stage, they do not immediately accept the diagnosis and tend to think that there has been a mistake. So they look for other doctors and retake tests. Stress is inevitable.

The fear of the unknown, suffering, distancing from people, real isolation, lack of future possibilities, child dependency frightens many parents who initially do not see the possibility of coping with the problem. The feeling of ambivalence, the mix of positive and negative feelings is initially constant (FREITAS, 2011, p.173).

In the third stage, parents feel sadness and/or anger when the diagnosis is confirmed. Anger at themselves for creating an "imperfect" child, or at loved ones who witnessed their "failure," or even at the child himself.

The loss of an imaginary child usually causes parents to feel frustration and sadness. Parents' self-esteem drops because of their inability to see a reflection of a healthy self-image in their child.

When parents receive support from family (grandparents, siblings, friends) and health professionals, especially psychologists, anxiety decreases and information about the pathology becomes clearer. Little by little they emotionally reorganize and feel more able to confront the situation, seeking to understand what really happened. The child is no longer perceived as a threat and begins to be seen as a fragile being in need of care.

While some couples come together in crisis situations, others do the opposite and distance themselves from each other (CANAVARRO & FONSCA, 2010). Because the crisis experienced by parents in the context of developmental defects has the power to both unite and divide.

In the equilibrium stage, parents feel less anxiety, have less intense emotional reactions, and gain greater confidence in their ability to care for their child (KLAUS and KENNEL, 1993). Adaptation is never complete, the authors caution. But there does seem to be some reduction in anxiety and improvement in self-perception as a caregiver.

The life history of each mother, father, and couple will influence the experience of each stage, as well as the duration of each stage and the possibility of reaching a stage of balance. The severity of the malformation, prognosis, and available resources (support, parental psychological structure) are factors that will influence the development of grief in parents (KROEFF, MAIA and LIMA, 2000, cited by GOMES, 2010).

In situations of malformations, death is a constant threat and parents feel overwhelmed by the fear of losing their child. It seems that both during pregnancy and after birth, parents, in defense, do not want to create a bond with the child because they are afraid of losing the child at any moment and thus do not create space in their minds for the child's mental constitution. child. If the parents' mind does not have the necessary readiness to form a coherent subject and if doubt, fear and overprotection are present in this relationship, the child's development may be impaired (JERUSALINSKI, 2002, cited by GOMES, 2010). This author introduces the concept of "funeral enclosure", that is, the second death, the result of the parents seeing, treating and caring for the child, that is, when the child, even if alive and spoken for, is seen and lived as dead. Nevertheless, according to this author, "parents need to be helped to realize that the worst thing that can happen in someone's life is that nothing happens to them" (JERUSALINSKI, 2002, cited by GOMES, 2007).

Parents often expect an accurate and objective prognosis. They ask the medical team many questions and feel overwhelmed and unhelpful by the news of the birth defect. The shock of the news also seems to make it difficult for parents to understand the diagnosis.

According to Moreira, Morsch, and Braga (2006, p. 159):

"Medicine is often expected to be accurate, typical of a science that is considered objective. In other words, when medical care is needed, it is considered an exact science capable of providing absolutely accurate provision and care. However, it is a branch of knowledge aimed at the study of personal health, which in itself makes it subjective. [...] Thus, it is clear that medicine cannot be viewed as a "crystal ball," although many families of newborns tend to believe this assumption. Also cause her surprise when she encounters a change in the baby's gait."

Regarding diagnosis, in a study of one hundred ninety-four mothers of infants with cleft spine, Klaus and Kennell (1993, p. 248) cite the following results:

"(...) two-thirds preferred to learn about the diagnosis as early as possible and were satisfied with the information they received about the defects. Any delay in receiving this information led to increased anxiety. They disapproved of receiving an unnecessarily discouraging picture on the one hand initially, and on the other hand disapproved of first minimizing the seriousness of the condition and then intensifying it."

We understand the difficulty and concern of physicians in informing parents about the effects of the malformation on the child's development, as each child is unique and responds differently to the proposed treatment. However, we could see from the parents' accounts that the severity of the prognosis causes them great anxiety and uncertainty.

Faced with a baby whose chance of survival is only 1%, parents find it difficult to prepare for the birth of this baby (do not provide shelter, do not create a physical and psychological space for the baby). On the contrary, they despair and avoid establishing a bond with the baby. According to a theoretical review conducted by Crowe (1996, cited by GOMES, 2007), parents of children with heart defects did not want to bond with the child because the child might not survive.

Therefore, as great as the need is for both doctors and parents to have an accurate prognosis, we believe that care must be taken to avoid adding negative fantasies to the parents' psyche. Parents also need to understand the limitations of medical science and stop viewing it as a "crystal ball."

The neonatal intensive care unit team can work on parent-baby contact, especially if the clinical condition of the baby does not allow the parents to hold the baby on their laps. Alternatives to contact with the baby can be offered to the parents by the team. Voice, gaze and touch are also forms of communication and play an important role in establishing the first bonds between parents and their baby.

Encouraging parents to participate in their baby's care may bring relief and reduce the feeling of incompetence they experience in the neonatal intensive care unit. This is because the presence of the medical team brings relief on the one hand, but can also make parents feel that they are not important to the baby at that moment (MOREIRA; BRAGA; MORSH, 2006).

According to Gomez (2003), "our role as health care providers is to help parents not just focus on the limitations and impossibilities of a given malformation, but to always recognize the possibilities and limitations of that particular child" (p. 13).

Some authors have agreed (Crespin, 2004; Gomes, 2007; Szejer, 1999) that psychological intervention with parents should begin as early as possible, that is, during prenatal care, to prevent possible psychological damage to the children. parents, for the child, and for the relationship. Ideally, once a malformation has been diagnosed, parents will be referred to psychotherapy as well as support groups.

According to Setubal (2004), psychological counseling was effective in helping parents whose children were diagnosed with malformations. It enabled parents to become active participants in the diagnostic and treatment process. This author also emphasized the importance of medical staff understanding the psychological implications that a diagnosis of a malformation can have on parents.

The process of grieving an "imaginary child" is long and difficult, with parents going through several stages as they try to adapt to the needs of their child with a malformation. The parents interviewed were confident in their ability to care for their child, especially after receiving guidance from the medical team and learning, for example, how to perform catheterization.

The birth of a child requires considerable effort on the part of parents to cope with the psychological and bodily changes that occur. The present study has shown that these changes are even more significant and fraught with suffering in the context of birth defects. Parents feel disoriented in the "moon world" when they discover that their child will be born with problems.

An overly disappointing prognosis causes parents a great deal of distress and prevents them from preparing for the birth of their baby. On the other hand, other studies have shown that parents also discourage minimizing the severity of the problem (KLAUS and KENNEL, 1993).

The inability to communicate created by a malformation does not preclude other forms of parent-baby relationships. It is interesting to consider the possibility that health care providers may offer these forms, if parents so desire, to facilitate their bonding with their child. In focusing on the limitations and impossibilities that accompany birth defects, both parents and the multidisciplinary team cannot overlook the opportunities for emotional interaction for that child. Care must be taken not to turn limitations into impossibilities. The development of a child with a malformation is fundamentally dependent on the proper conduct of treatment processes, both medical and psychological, especially in the postpartum period.

The emotional support offered by health professionals and psychotherapy is important because it helps parents in the process of bonding with their child and allows parents to become more active and confident in their ability to care for their child and themselves.

BIBLIOGRAPHIC REFERENCES

AMORIM, Melania Maria Ramos de et al. Impact of congenital malformations on perinatal and neonatal mortality in a teaching maternity hospital in Recife. Rev. Bras. Maternal and child health. Recife, 2012. Available in: http://dx.doi.org/10.1590/S1519-38292006000500003. Accessed: 02.12.12 .

BELFORT, Paulo; BRAGA, Antonio; FREIRE, Nazare Serra. Uterine arteriovenous malformation after gestational trophoblastic disease. Brazilian reverend gynecologic obstetrician. São Paulo, vol.28, no.2, pp.112-121, February 2006.

BRAZIL. RDC Regulation No. 344 of December 13, 2002. Technical regulation on the fortification of wheat and corn flour with iron and folic acid. Official Gazette of the Union, Brasilia, December 18, 2002.

BRASELTON, Berry T.; KREMER, Bertrand G. First relationships. São Paulo: Martins Fontes, 1992.

BOWLBY, John. A secure base. Porto Alegre: Ed Artes Medicas, 1989.

BYDLOWSKI, Monique. The pregnant woman's inner gaze: psychic transparency and representation. In: New perspectives on pregnancy and children under 3 years of age: perinatal health, education and child development. Brasilia: LGE Editora, 2002.

CANAVARRO, Maria Cristina and FONSCA, Ana. Parents' reactions to the perinatal diagnosis of a congenital anomaly in their child and implications for health professionals' intervention. Psychology, Health and Disease. Coimbra, vol. 11, n. 2, c.283 297, 2010.

CRESPEN, Graciela Culliere. Early clinic: the birth of man. São Paulo: Casa do Psicologo, 2004.

DE ANDRADE, Maria Auxiliadora Gomes. Becoming a father, becoming a mother: the process of parenthood. In: New perspectives on pregnancy and children under 3 years of age: perinatal health, education and child development. Brasilia: LGE

Editora, 2002.

FREITAS, Ghislaine Vaz S. de. 10 psychological reactions of parents to their "special" child. In: Myelomeningocele.

GAIVA, Maria Aparecida Muñoz; MODES, Priscilla Shirley Siniak. The child with cleft spine: basics of nursing care. In: Proc. Health of children and adolescents, vol. 2. Porto Alegre: Artmed Editora, 2010.

GOLSE, Bernard. What we have learned from infants. In: New perspectives on pregnancy and children under 3 years of age: perinatal health, education and child development. Brasilia: LGE Editora, 2002.

GOMEZ, Alyn Grill. Child malformations and motherhood: the impact of brief parent-child psychotherapy on mothers' perceptions. Doctoral dissertation. Federal University of Rio Grande do Sul, 2007.

JERUSALINSKY, Juliet. Chronicle of a child whose death was announced - an intervention to bring the subject to the brink of death. In: BERNARD INO, Leda and ROHENKOL, Claudia. (Org.) The infant and modernity: clinical-theoretical approaches. São Paulo: Casa do Psicologo, 2002.

CLAUS, Marshall H.; KENNELL, John H. Parent/child: the formation of attachment. Porto Alegre: Ed Artes Medicas, 1993.

CREFF, C.; MAYA, C.; and LIMA, C. Mourning the ugly child. Rev. Femina, 28, 395-396, 2000.

LEBOVICH, Serge. The infant, the mother and the psychoanalyst. Porto Alegre: Ed. Artes Medicas, 1987.

MALDONADO, Maria Teresa. Psychology of pregnancy: labor and postpartum. São Paulo: Ed Saraiva, 1997.

MOREIRA, Maria Elizabeth Lopez; BRAGA, Nina de Almeida; MORSH, Denise Streit.

When life begins differently: a baby and his family in the neonatal intensive care unit. Rio de Janeiro: Fiocruz, 2006.

PICCININININI, Cesar Augusto et al. Paternal involvement during pregnancy. Psychol. reflex. Crit. Porto Alegre, Vol. 17, No. 3, 2004 Available at: http://dx.doi.org/10.1590/S0102-79722004000300003 . Accessed 10/11/12.

RAMIREZ, Vera Regina Ronelt; SCHNEIDER, Michelle Scheffel. Returning to some concepts of attachment theory: behavior or representation? Psych: Theor. and research. Brasilia, vol. 26, no. March 1. 2010. Available at < http://www.scielo.com.brhttp://dx.doi.org/10.1590/S0102-37722010000100004 . Accessed: 05.10.12.

SETUBAL, M.S. et al. Psychological reactions to pregnancy complicated by fetal malformations. Program of Fetal Medicine (PMF), Department of Tocogynecology, Faculty of Health Sciences, State University of Campinas (UNICAMP), pp. 1-12, 2004. Available at:
http://www.barini.med.br/publicacao . Date of reference: 01.06.2013.

SOUZA, Alex Sandro Rolland, et al. al. Spina bifida: current concepts. Revista Femina, vol. 35, no. 7, 453-460, July 2007 Available at: http://www.febrasgo.com.br/extras/downloads/revistaFeminaZip/2007-35-7/Femina35(7)p455-62.pdf . Accessed: 28.05.2013.

STERN, Daniel. Constellation of motherhood. Porto Alegre: Ed. Artes Medicas, 1997. The interpersonal world of the child. Porto Alegre: Ed Artes Medicas, 1992.

SUASCUNA, Ana Maria Vilar. Influence of prenatal diagnosis on the formation of possible psychopathologies of the infant-parental oz. In: Psychoanalysis and clinic with infants: symptoms, treatment and interdisciplinary approach in early childhood. São Paulo: Language Institute, 2010.

SEYER, Miriam. Words to be born: psychoanalytic listening in motherhood. São Paulo: Casa do Psicologo, 1999.

SEYER, Miriam. A psychoanalytic approach to pregnancy and childbirth. In: New perspectives on pregnancy and children under 3 years of age: perinatal health, education and child development. Brasilia: LGE Editora, 2002.

WINNICOTT, Donald Wood. From pediatrics to psychoanalysis. Rio de Janeiro: Edited by Francisco Alvesa, 1978.

ZORNIG, Sylvia Maria Abu-Jamrah. Becoming a father, becoming a mother: the process of constructing parenthood. Journal Tempo Psicanalitico. Rio de Janeiro, vol. 42.2, pp. 453-470, 2010 г. Available at: http://xa.yimg.com/kq/groups/2413 7146/422807075/name/O+processo+de+constru%C3%A7%C3%A3o+da+parentalidade.pdf. Date of circulation: 05.10.2012.

Publishers:

Flavio Freinkel Rodriguez.
Associate Professor of Medicine at UFRJ
Master's and Doctor of Surgery UFRJ
Member of the Brazilian Academy of Neurosurgery.
Postdoctoral fellow in neurosurgery at René Descartes University.
Hospitaller Center Saint-Anne, Paris, France.

Eliete Botelho Cardoso
Master's student of the Professional Master's Program "Perinatal Health"
UFRW Maternity Hospital
Specialist in integrated maternal and child health care
UFRW Maternity Hospital
Social worker at Sociedade Universitaria Augusto Motta

Co-authors:
Joana Ayla Donzelli
Specialist in integrated maternal and child health care
Maternity Hospital - UFRJ
Specialist in Clinical Psychology, Phenomenology - IFEN
Psychology - Santa Ursula University
Clinical psychology and breastfeeding counseling - Espaco Ama Psychology

Mauricio Moscovici (In memoriam)

A full professor of anatomy at UFRJ
FFU Professor Emeritus.
Professor Emeritus of the Campos Faculty of Medicine
Honorary Fellow of the American Association of Anatomy.

Torquil Diniz Javier de Brito.
Neurosurgery at the Federal Hospital of Ipanema
Member of the Brazilian Society of Neurosurgery

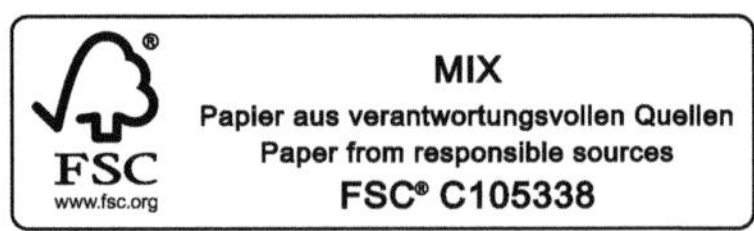

Printed by Books on Demand GmbH, Norderstedt / Germany